Simple Low Sodium & Low Fat Recipes to Cook Heart Healthy Recipes

in 30 minutes or less

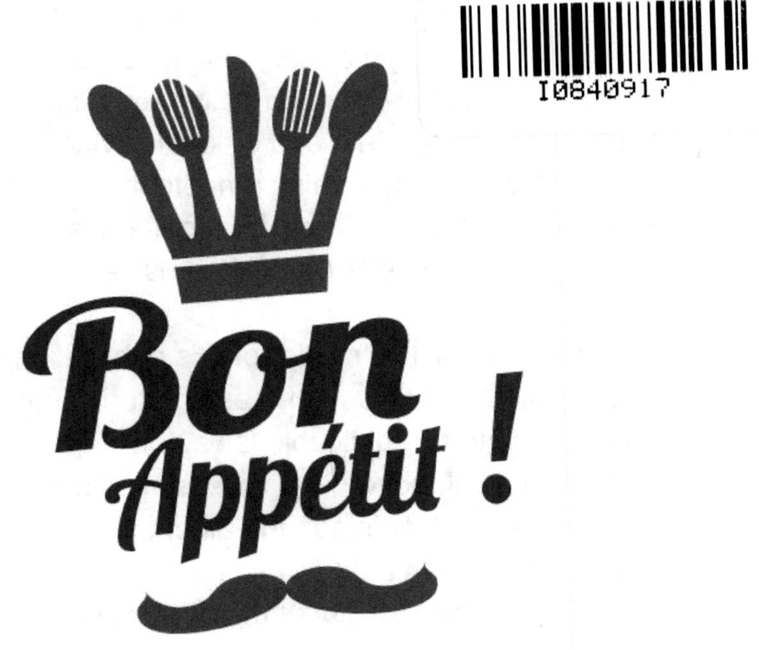

Table of Contents

Frequent Measurement Conversions

Liquid Measures

1 gal = 4 qt = 8 pt = 16 cups = 128 fl oz
½ gal = 2 qt = 4 pt = 8 cups = 64 fl oz
¼ gal = 1 qt = 2 pt = 4 cups = 32 fl oz
½ qt = 1 pt = 2 cups = 16 fl oz
¼ qt = ½ pt = 1 cup = 8 fl oz

Dry Measures

1 cup = 16 Tbsp = 48 tsp = 250ml
¾ cup = 12 Tbsp = 36 tsp = 175ml
⅔ cup = 10 ⅔ Tbsp = 32 tsp = 150ml
½ cup = 8 Tbsp = 24 tsp = 125ml
⅓ cup = 5 ⅓ Tbsp = 16 tsp = 75ml
¼ cup = 4 Tbsp = 12 tsp = 50ml
⅛ cup = 2 Tbsp = 6 tsp = 30ml
1 Tbsp = 3 tsp = 15ml

Dash or Pinch or Speck = less than ⅛ tsp

Quickies

1 fl oz = 30 ml
1 oz = 28.35 g
1 lb = 16 oz (454 g)
1 kg = 2.2 lb
1 quart = 2 pints

U.S.	Canadian
¼ tsp	1.25 mL
½ tsp	2.5 mL
1 tsp	5 mL
1 Tbl	15 mL
¼ cup	50 mL
⅓ cup	75 mL
½ cup	125 mL
⅔ cup	150 mL
¾ cup	175 mL
1 cup	250 mL
1 quart	1 liter

Recipe Abbreviations

Cup = c or C
Fluid = fl
Gallon = gal
Ounce = oz
Package = pkg
Pint = pt
Pound = lb or #
Quart = qt
Square = sq
Tablespoon = T or Tbl
   or TBSP or TBS
Teaspoon = t or tsp

*Some measurements were rounded

Fahrenheit (°F) to Celcius (°C)

$°C = (°F - 32) \times 5/9$

Fahrenheit	Celcius
32 °F	0 °C
40 °F	4 °C
140 °F	60 °C
150 °F	65 °C
160 °F	70 °C
225 °F	107 °C
250 °F	121 °C
275 °F	135 °C
300 °F	150 °C
325 °F	165 °C
350 °F	177 °C
375 °F	190 °C
400 °F	205 °C
425 °F	220 °C
450 °F	230 °C
475 °F	245 °C
500 °F	260 °C

OVEN TEMPERATURES

WARMING: 200 °F
VERY SLOW: 250 °F - 275 °F
SLOW: 300 °F - 325 °F
MODERATE: 350 °F - 375 °F
HOT: 400 °F - 425 °F
VERY HOT: 450 °F - 475 °F

Introduction

Heart Health is that every American and over the world citizen should be concerned about. Different heart diseases are one of the main death reasons for both men and women. Moreover, cardiovascular diseases often called as "the silent killer" because it cannot be any warning signs before a heart attack strikes.

Fortunately, heart health is under your control. Surely, there're many factors that cannot be changed, such as age or family history, but you can reduce risk of heart attacks choosing a healthy way of life.

Unfortunately, many people do not use healthy habits for various reasons. Some do not have enough time, some do not have enough knowledge, for some people it's too hard. However, you need to understand that your healthy lifestyle is the best protection against heart diseases, so a healthy way of life is the simplest way to live a long happy life.

Properly formulated diet is one of the easiest and most effective ways to reduce heart diseases attacks. Many people do not know what meals to eat in order to keep the heart and blood vessels healthy. That is why I created this book, which contains delicious, easy, and at the same time useful heart healthy recipes for two that will allow you to eat properly, and also reduce the risk of cardiovascular diseases.

12 Useful tips to minimize risk of heart healthy diseases

Eat heart healthy meals. Make fruit, vegetables, fish, and whole grains the main in your diet.

1. **Limit** sodium, saturated fats and sweets.

2. **Be active.** Try to walk at least 10 000 steps per day.

3. **Control your blood sugar.** Blood glucose should be less than 100 mg/dL

4. **Control your cholesterol.** Total cholesterol should be less than 200 mg/dL

5. **Control your blood pressure.** Try to keep your numbers below 120/80 mm Hg

6. **Live smoke-free**

7. **Drink more green tea.** It reduces the risk of heart attack.

8. **Reach for vitamin D.** Nearly 75% of heart patients are deficient in Vitamin D.

9. **Have an optimistic outlook.**

10. **Keep calm.** Try to find 30 minutes per day for relaxation techniques such as deep breathing or meditation.

11. **More muscle – less fat.** Do more physique exercises.

Low Calories Roasted Salmon with Beans & Tomatoes

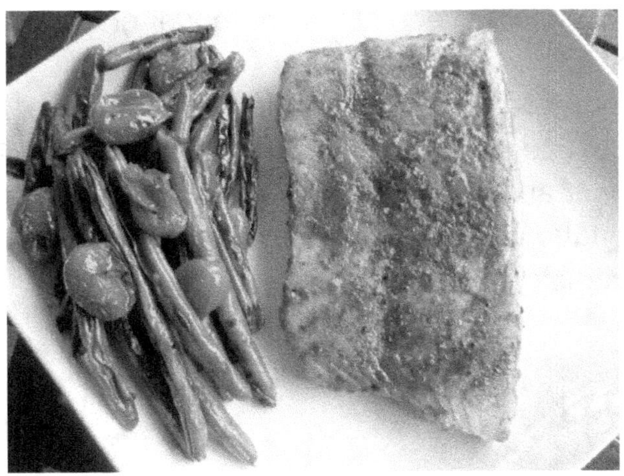

- Prep time: 15 minutes
- Cook time: 20 minutes
- Calories: 304

Ingredients

- 1 large skinless salmon fillet
- 4 clove garlic
- 1 lb. green beans
- 1 pt. grape tomatoes
- 1/2 c. pitted kalamata olives
- 2 tbsp. olive oil
- kosher salt
- Pepper to taste

Directions

1. Preheat oven to 415 F.

2. In the large bowl mix together the garlic, beans, tomatoes, olives, with 1 tablespoon oil and 1/4 teaspoon pepper. Replace to the baking sheet and roast until the vegetables are tender and beginning to brown.
3. Meanwhile, heat the remaining tablespoon oil in a large skillet over medium heat. Season the salmon with pepper and cook until golden brown and opaque throughout, 4 to 5 minutes per side. Serve with the vegetables.

Fusilli with Broccoli Topping

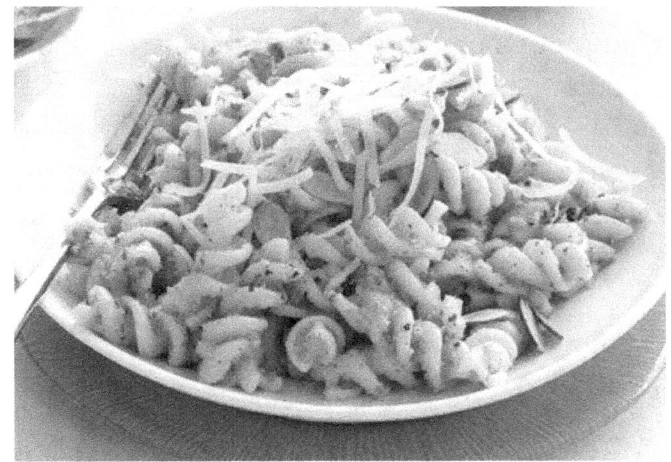

- Prep time: 10 minutes
- Cook time: 15 minutes
- Calories: 340

Ingredients

- 6 oz. fusilli pasta
- 6 oz. frozen broccoli florets
- 1-2 clove garlic
- 1/4 cup fresh basil leaves or 1 tbsp dried basil
- 3 tbsp. olive oil
- 1 tbsp. grated lemon zest
- Parmesan cheese, grated (if desired)

Directions

1. Cook the pasta according to package directions. Reserve 1/2 cup of the cooking liquid, drain the pasta, and return it to the pot.
2. Meanwhile, in a microwave-safe bowl, combine the broccoli, garlic, and 1/2 cup water. Cover and cook on

high, stirring once halfway through, until the broccoli is tender, 5 to 6 minutes. Transfer the mixture (liquid included) to a food processor. Add the basil, oil, zest, and purée until smooth.

3. Toss the pasta with the pesto and 1/4 cup of the reserved liquid. Sprinkle with grated Parmesan cheese if desired.

Delicious Chicken Stir-Fry with Rice

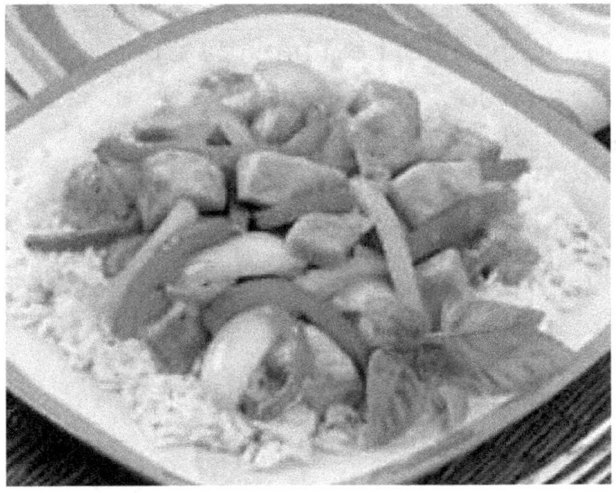

- Prep time: 15 minutes
- Cook time: 30 minutes
- Calories: 432

Ingredients

- 1/2 pound chicken breasts, boneless and skinless
- 1/2 cup brown rice
- 1/4 cup apricot preserves
- 1 tbsp vinegar
- 1 tsp ginger, grated
- A pinch of red pepper flakes
- 3 tbsp olive oil
- 1 medium-sized carrot
- 1/4 pound snow peas

Directions

1. Cook the rice according to package directions.

2. While rice is cooking, in a medium mixing bowl combine apricots, vinegar, grated ginger, pepper flacks and some water. Set aside.
3. Cut lengthwise chicken breasts. Preheat the skillet oven medium-high heat and roast chicken until golden brown, for about 3-5 minutes per side. Transfer to a plate.
4. Add chopped carrots, snow peas and some oil to the skillet and cook for 2-3 minutes, stirring occasionally. Return the chicken fillets to the skillet, pour over the apricot mixture and cook for another 3-4 minutes until vegetables become tender.
5. Serve with rice and enjoy!

Tilapia with Rice, Pineapple and Cucumber

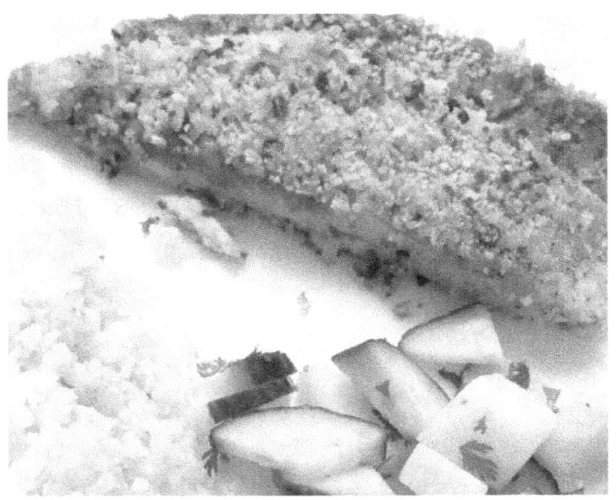

- Prep time: 15 minutes
- Cook time: 20 minutes
- Calories: 370

Ingredients

- 2 medium-sized tilapia fillets
- 1 cup long-grain white rice
- 2 tbsp. fresh lime juice
- 1 tbsp. grated ginger
- 2 tsp. honey
- 2 tbsp. olive oil
- 1 jalapeño pepper, chopped
- 1/2 small pineapple, chopped
- 1 small English cucumber, chopped
- Pepper to taste

Directions

1. Firstly, cook the rice according to package directions.
2. Meanwhile, in a large bowl, whisk together the lime juice, ginger, honey, olive oil and some pepper. Toss with jalapeño, pineapple and cucumber.
3. Heat the remaining tsp oil in a large nonstick skillet over medium heat. Season the tilapia with pepper and cook until golden brown and cooked through, 1 to 3 minutes per side. Serve the fish with the rice and vegetable mixture.

Delicious Sugar Snap Peas and Radish Salad

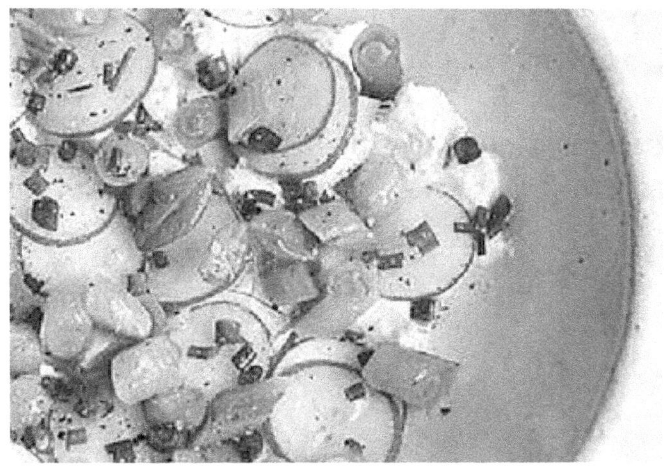

- Prep time: 10 minutes
- Cook time: 10 minutes
- Calories: 135

Ingredients

- 1 pound sugar snap peas
- 12 small radishes
- 1/2 medium ripe avocado
- 2 tbsp. apple-cider vinegar
- 1 tbsp. fresh lemon juice
- 1/2 tsp. Dijon mustard
- 1/2 tsp. salt
- 1/2 tsp. Freshly ground pepper
- 1/4 tsp. ground coriander
- 3 tbsp olive oil

Directions

1. In a large bowl, combine sugar snap peas and
    radishes. Set aside.
2. In a blender or the bowl of a food processor, combine
    avocado, vinegar, lemon juice, mustard, salt, pepper,
    and coriander. Gradually add oil, blending until mixture
    is a smooth purée. If needed add couple tbsp water.
3. Toss salad with dressing to coat and serve
    immediately.

Heart Healthy Bean Burrito Bowl

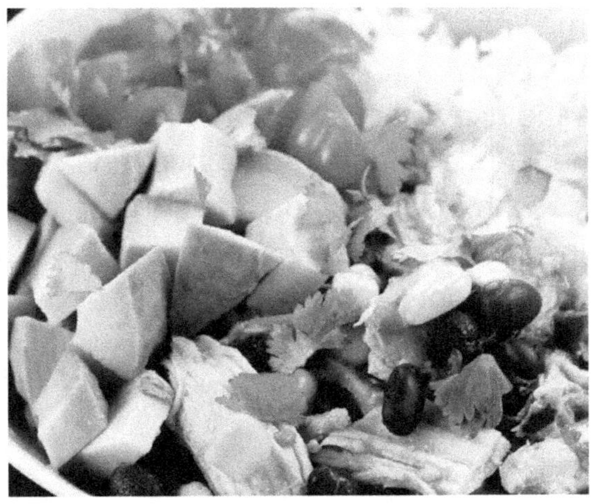

- Prep time: 20 minutes
- Cook time: 25 minutes
- Calories: 312

Ingredients

- 1 cup cooked brown rice
- 1 small avocado
- 1/2 can black beans
- 2 tbsp fresh lime juice
- 2 tbsp olive oil
- 1/2 tsp. ground cumin
- 1/4 head romaine lettuce
- 1 tbsp dried cilantro
- 5 cherry tomatoes, cut
- 1/2 small red onion
- 2 tbsp low-fat sour cream
- Tortilla chips, lime wedges for dressing
- Hot sauce to taste

Directions

1. In a small mixing bowl, whisk together the lime juice, oil, and cumin.
2. Divide the rice and beans among serving bowls. Top with the lettuce, cilantro, tomatoes, and avocado.
3. Sprinkle with the red onion, then drizzle with the dressing. Serve with sour cream, tortilla chips, lime wedges, and hot sauce, if desired.

Chickpea and Red Pepper Soup with Quinoa

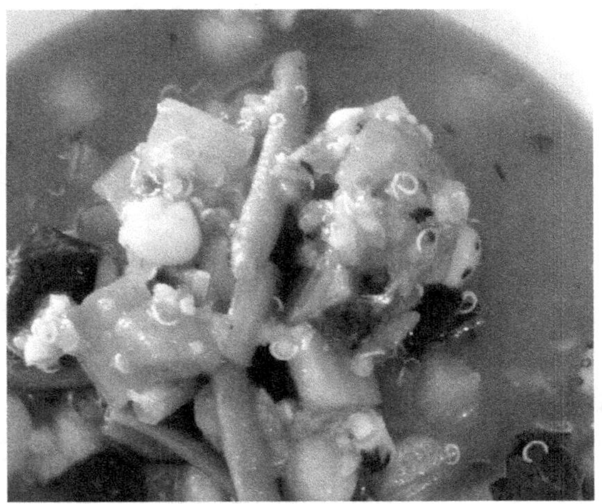

- Prep time: 20 minutes
- Cook time: 25 minutes
- Calories: 384

Ingredients

- 1/4 cup uncooked quinoa
- 2 tbsp olive oil
- 1 small onion, chopped
- 1 small carrot, chopped
- 1 stalk celery, chopped
- 2 garlic cloves, minced
- 1 tsp smoked paprika
- A pinch of salt and pepper
- 1 medium yellow bell pepper
- 1 medium red bell pepper
- 1 can low-sodium chickpeas
- 1 cup low-sodium vegetable broth

- 1 tbsp red wine vinegar
- Chopped fresh parsley for garnish

Directions

1. Cook the quinoa according to package directions.
2. While cooking heat the oil in a Dutch oven or large heavy-bottomed pot. Add the onion, carrot, and celery and cook, covered, stirring occasionally, for 6 minutes.
3. Then, add garlic, paprika, season with salt and pepper and cook, stirring, for 1 minute. Add bell peppers and cook for another 5 minutes.
4. Add the chickpeas, broth, and 1 cup water and bring to a boil. Reduce heat and simmer until the vegetables are tender, 5 to 8 minutes. Stir in the vinegar and cooked quinoa. Serve topped with parsley, if desired.

Sweet and Spicy Glazed Salmon with Delicious Rice

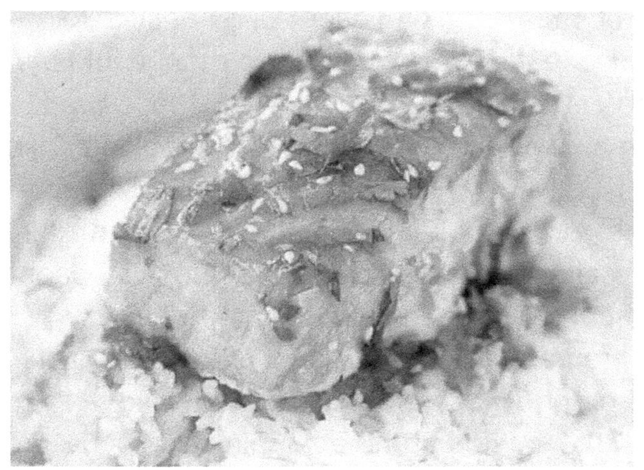

- Prep time: 15 minutes
- Cook time: 25 minutes
- Calories: 498

Ingredients

- 2 salmon fillets
- 1/2 cup long-grain white rice
- 5 tbsp sliced almonds
- 1 small orange
- 1/4 cup hot pepper jelly
- A pinch of salt and pepper to taste
- Freshly chopped parsley

Directions

1. Heat oven to 390 F. Cook the rice according to package directions.

2. While rice cooking, spread the almonds on a baking
    sheet and roast until light golden brown, for 5 minutes.
    Then transfer to a bowl. Heat broiler. Line a broiler-
    proof rimmed baking sheet with nonstick foil.
3. Squeeze the juice from half an orange into a small bowl
    and get 2 tablespoons juice. Add the jelly and whisk to
    combine. Place the salmon on the baking sheet,
    season with 1/2 teaspoon each salt and pepper, and
    roast for 5 minutes. Spoon half the jelly mixture over
    the salmon and broil until the salmon is opaque
    throughout, 2 to 5 minutes more.
4. Cut remain half of the orange into 1/2-inch pieces. Fold
    the oranges, almonds, and parsley into the rice. Serve
    with the salmon and the remaining jelly mixture.

Black Bean and Avocado Salsa

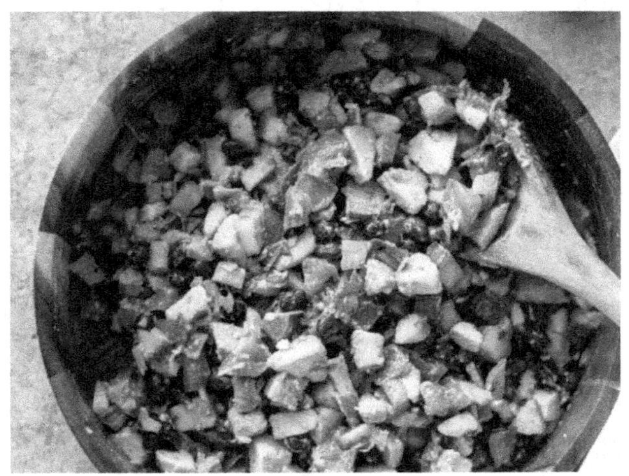

- Prep time: 10 minutes
- Cook time: 15 minutes
- Calories: 143

Ingredients

- 1/2 can black beans
- 1 garlic clove, minced
- 1 jalapeño pepper
- 1 small onion, chopped
- Salt and pepper to taste
- 2 scallions
- 2 tbsp. fresh lime juice
- 1 tbsp. olive oil
- 1 medium-sized avocado
- 1 tsp dried cilantro

Directions

1. In a large bowl, combine chopped jalapeño, garlic, onion, and season with salt and pepper.

2. Add beans, scallions, lime juice, and oil and toss to combine. Fold in the avocado and cilantro.
3. Serve and enjoy!

Quinoa Bowl with Red Pepper, Green Beans, and Red Onion

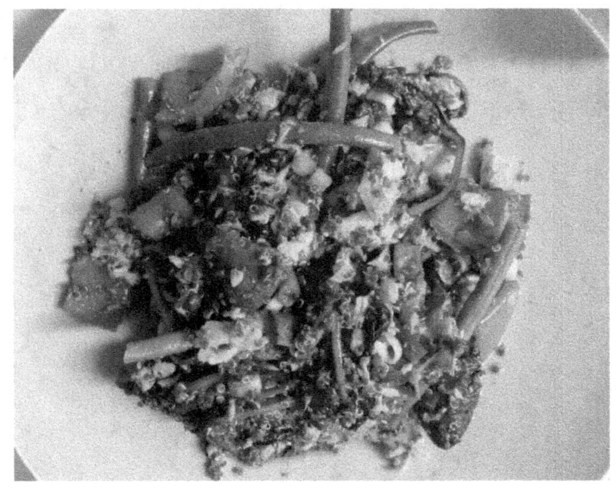

- Prep time: 10 minutes
- Cook time: 15 minutes
- Calories: 154

Ingredients

- 1/2 cup uncooked quinoa
- 1/4 tsp salt
- 1/4 tsp pepper
- 1 jarred roasted red pepper
- 2 oz green beans
- 1 small red onion, chopped
- 1 tbsp olive oil
- 2 tsp red wine vinegar

Directions

1. Place quinoa in a medium saucepan and pour with 2 cups water. Bring to a boil, add some salt, then reduce

heat and simmer, covered, until all the liquid has absorbed, nearly 10 minutes.

2. While cooking, in a large bowl, whisk together oil and vinegar, season with salt and pepper, stir to combine. Add red peppers, beans, and onion and toss to combine. Add the prepared quinoa mix evenly. Serve.

Avocados with Creamy Crab Salad

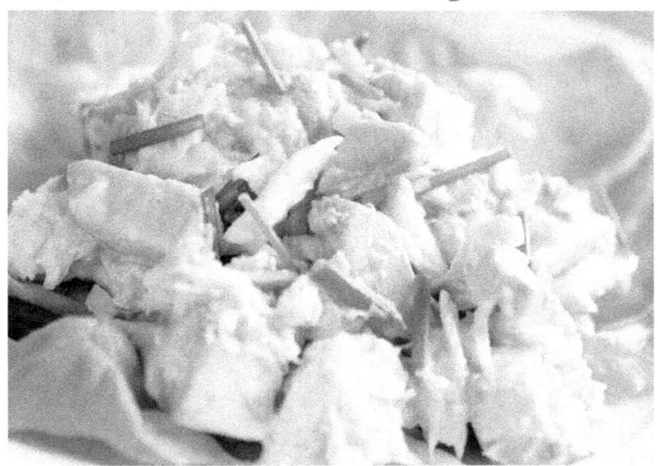

- Prep time: 3 minutes
- Cook time: 5 minutes
- Calories: 519

Ingredients

- 3 firm ripped avocados
- 1 tbsp grated lemon zest
- 4 tbsp fresh lemon juice
- 1 pound lump crab meat
- 1/4 cup radishes, diced
- 4 tbsp light mayonnaise
- 1 tsp dried basil

Directions

1. Cut 2 avocados in half. Chop remaining avocado in 1/2-inch dice. Sprinkle 2 tablespoons of the lemon juice over halved and diced avocados.

2. In large bowl combine diced avocado, lemon zest, the
    remaining 2 tablespoons lemon juice, crab meat,
    radishes, mayonnaise, and basil, tossing lightly.
3. Spoon mixture into the cut halves of avocado.
4. Serve with grilled or toasted pita bread if desired.

Horseradish Salmon Cakes

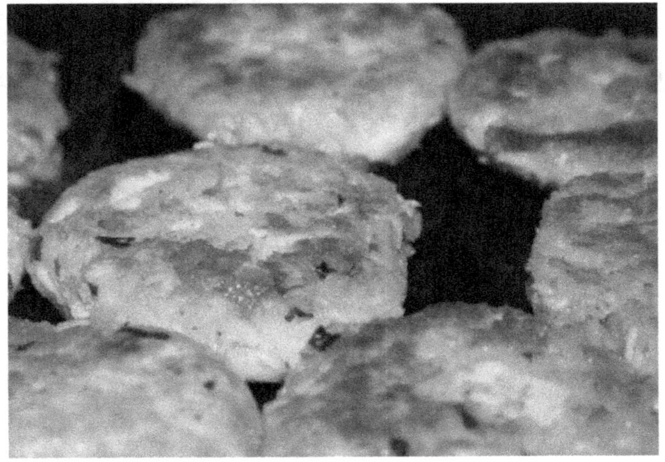

- Prep time: 15 minutes
- Cook time: 20 minutes
- Calories: 301

Ingredients

- 2 medium-sized salmon fillets
- 1 tbsp prepared horseradish
- 1 tbsp Dijon mustard
- 5 tbsp Panko bread crumbs
- 2 tbsp olive oil
- 2 tbsp fat-less Greek yogurt
- 1 tbsp fresh lemon juice
- 1 small English cucumber
- A bunch watercress
- A pinch of salt and pepper to taste

Directions

1. In a food processor blend the salmon, horseradish,
    mustard, salt, and pepper until coarsely chopped. Stir in
    bread crumbs and form the mixture into 8 patties.
2. Heat 1 tablespoon oil in a large nonstick skillet over
    medium heat. Cook the patties until brown, 2 minutes
    per side.
3. In a large bowl, whisk together the yogurt, lemon juice,
    remaining oil. Season with salt and pepper. Add the
    cucumbers and toss to coat; fold in the watercress.
    Serve with the patties.

Balsamic Chicken with Apple, Lentil, and Spinach Salad

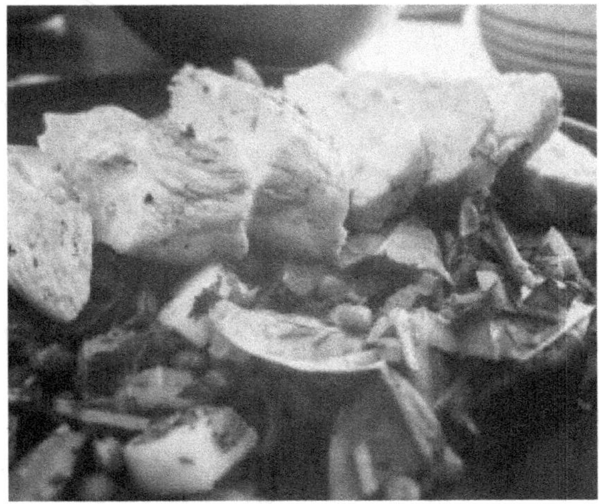

- Prep time: 15 minutes
- Cook time: 20 minutes
- Calories: 387

Ingredients

- 1 large chicken breast, boneless and skinless
- 1 scallions
- 1 small green apple
- 1 stalk celery
- 1 tbsp fresh lemon juice
- 1/2 can lentils
- 1 cup baby spinach
- 1/4 cup fresh flat-leaf parsley
- 3 tbsp olive oil
- A pinch of salt and pepper to taste
- 2 tbsp balsamic vinegar

Directions

1. Heat 1 tablespoon oil in a large skillet over medium heat. Season the chicken with salt and pepper and cook until golden brown, nearly 6-7 minutes each side. Remove from heat and add the vinegar. Turn the chicken to coat.
2. While cooking, in a large bowl, place scallions, apple, celery, lemon juice, 1 tablespoon oil, season with salt and pepper. Fold in the lentils, spinach and parsley (if desired) and serve with the chicken.

Heart Healthy Minestrone Soup

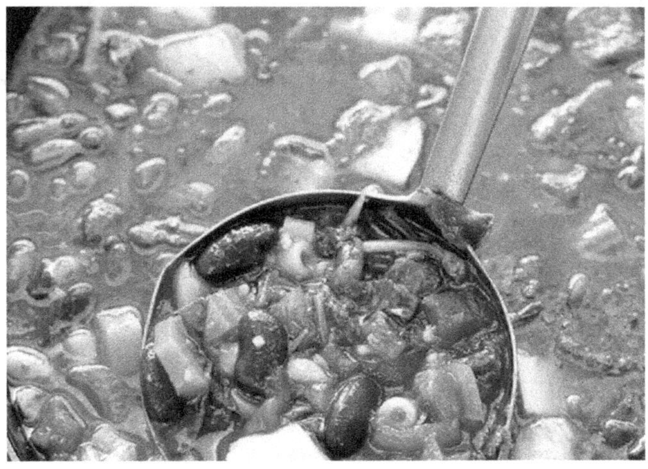

- Prep time: 10 minutes
- Cook time: 20 minutes
- Calories: 286

Ingredients

- 1/2 pound asparagus, trimmed and cut into 1-inch pieces
- 1/2 can white beans, rinsed
- 2 tbsp olive oil
- 1 stalk celery, chopped
- 1 leek (white and light green parts only), finely chopped
- 1 small onion, chopped
- 2 medium-sized potatoes, cut in 1/2-inch pieces
- 3 sprigs fresh thyme
- 3 oz. sugar snap peas, halved
- Some freshly chopped dill for serving
- A pinch of salt and pepper to taste

Directions

1. Heat oil in a Dutch oven on medium. Add celery, leeks, onion, season with salt and pepper and cook, covered, stirring occasionally, until tender.
2. Add potatoes, thyme, and 6 cups water and bring to a boil, then simmer 8 minutes. Add asparagus and simmer 2 minutes.
3. Add sugar snap peas and beans and simmer until vegetables are just tender, 3 to 4 minutes more. Discard thyme sprigs. Sprinkle soup with dill and serve.

Delicious Tortilla Fish Sticks with Purple Cabbage Slaw

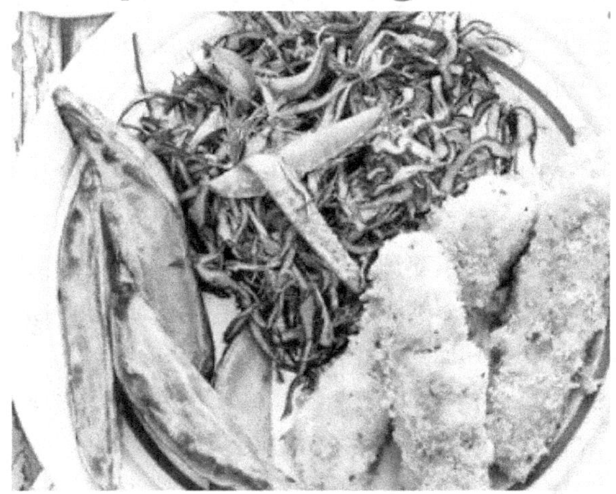

- Prep time: 5 minutes
- Cook time: 25 minutes
- Calories: 376

Ingredients

- 1 pound tilapia fillets
- 1/2 small red cabbage, cored and finely chopped
- 1 small orange
- 3 tbsp fresh lime juice
- 1 tsp sugar
- 5 tbsp sour cream
- 1 medium-sized carrot, grated
- 1 small red onion, chopped
- 2 cups tortilla chips, crushed
- 1 tsp dried cilantro
- 1/4 tsp salt
- 1/4 tsp pepper

Directions

1. Heat oven to 425°F. Take the large bowl and grate 1 tsp zest from orange into it. Squeeze in juice (about 1/3 cup). Whisk in lime juice, add sugar, salt and pepper to taste, whisk in sour cream.
2. Transfer 1/2 cup mixture to a shallow bowl. Add carrots, onion, and cabbage to the large bowl and let sit.
3. Meanwhile, line a rimmed baking sheet with foil. Cut tilapia into large chunks. Dip fish in reserved sour cream mixture and then in crushed chips, pressing gently to help them adhere.
4. Transfer fish chunks to the baking sheet and cook until light golden brown for about 8-10 minutes. Fold cilantro into slaw and serve with fish.

Spaghetti Squash and Chickpea Sauté

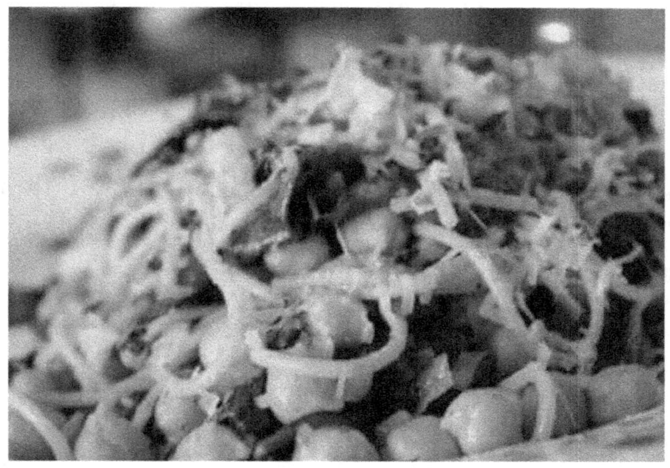

- Prep time: 5 minutes
- Cook time: 15 minutes
- Calories: 289

Ingredients

- 1 pound spaghetti squash
- 1 small red onion, finely chopped
- 3 tbsp fresh lemon juice
- 2 tbsp olive oil
- 1 garlic clove, minced
- 1/2 can chickpeas, rinsed
- 1/2 cup fresh flat-leaf parsley, chopped
- 2 oz crumbled feta
- Ground black pepper to taste

Directions

1. Prepare spaghetti squash and halve with large knife. Place them on a large paper sheet and microwave on high for 5-7 minutes until tender. Transfer cooked spaghetti to a large bowl.
2. Meanwhile, in a small mixing bowl toss onion, lemon juice and season with salt and pepper.
3. Sprinkle a non-stick skillet with 1 tbsp olive oil and toss minced garlic. Cook until golden brown. Add rinsed chickpeas and cook for couple minutes. Add spaghetti squash and 1 tablespoon olive oil.
4. Top with crumbled feta and serve.

Cod Fillets with Potatoes and Bacon

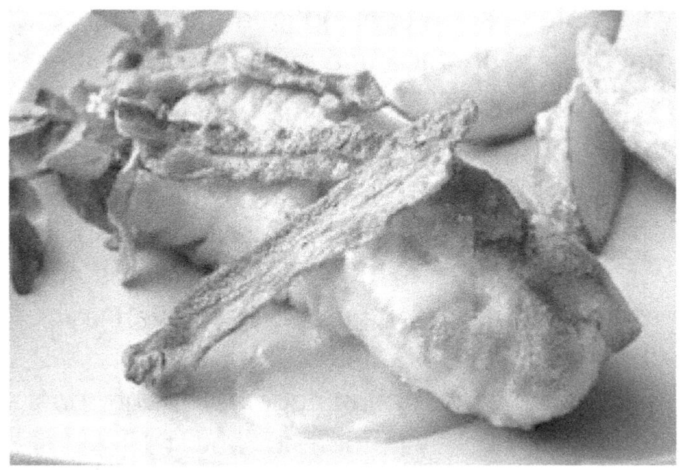

- Prep time: 15 minutes
- Cook time: 15 minutes
- Calories: 415

Ingredients

- 2 large cod fillets (1 inch thick)
- 2 slices bacon, cut into 1/2-inch pieces
- 1/2 pound small potatoes, halved
- 1 medium red onion cut into 1/2 inch lengthwise
- 1 tbsp. mayonnaise
- 1 tbsp. Dijon mustard
- 5 tbsp panko bread crumbs
- 1 tbsp olive oil
- 1 tbsp Thyme leaves
- Salt and black pepper

Directions

1. Preheat the oven to 450 F. Place potatoes and onions
    in the center of a baking sheet and place bacon on top.
    Roast for 10 minutes.
2. While potatoes are cooking, in a medium mixing bowl
    combine mayonnaise and mustard. In another bowl,
    combine Panko with oil, then sprinkle with thyme.
    Season fish with salt and pepper, then spread with
    mayonnaise mixture and sprinkle with Panko.
3. Remove the baking sheet from the oven and reduce
    oven temperature to 400 F. Toss potatoes and onion
    mixture together, then spread in an even layer,
    arranging potatoes cut side down.
4. Nestle fish pieces among vegetables and roast until fish
    is tender and lightly golden, for about 10-12 minutes.

Slow Cooker Pork with Spinach Rice

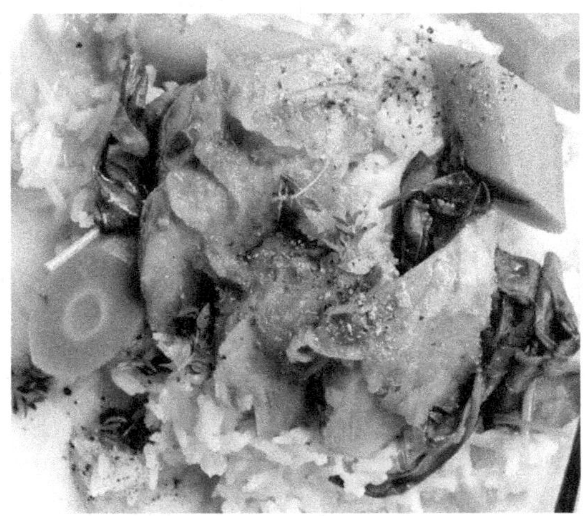

- Prep time: 15 minutes
- Cook time: 2 hours
- Calories: 475

Ingredients

- 1/2 pound pork tenderloin
- 1/2 cup long-grain white rice
- 1 small green apple
- 1 small onion
- 1 tbsp flour
- 1 cup baby spinach
- 2 large carrots (about 1/2 pound), cut into 2-inch pieces
- 2 tbsp Dijon mustard
- 2 tbsp honey
- 1 tbsp low-sodium soy sauce
- 4 sprigs fresh thyme, plus extra leaves for serving
- Salt and pepper to taste

Directions

1. Chop apple and onion and add to a slow cooker bowl. Toss with the flour and then add carrots.
2. In another mixing bowl combine mustard, honey and soy sauce. Cut the pork into 2 pieces and place to a slow cooker. Pour with the mustard mixture and mix to combine. Sprinkle with salt and pepper and add some thyme on top.
3. Secure the lid and cook until carrots are tender, about 2 hours.
4. Meanwhile, cook rice according the package directions.
5. Open the lid and discard the thyme. Transfer the meat to the cutting board and slice it. Add baby spinach to the slow cooker and stir to combine well. Serve sliced pork with rice and veggies, sprinkle with some fresh dill or cilantro if desired.

Amazing Pork and Vegetable Stir-Fry

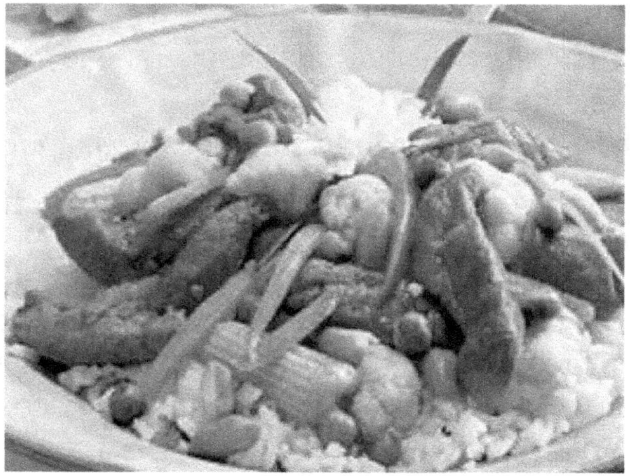

- Prep time: 30 minutes
- Cook time: 30 minutes
- Calories: 359

Ingredients

- 1/2 cup long-grain white rice
- 1/2 pound pork
- 2 tbsp hoisin sauce
- 1 tbsp fresh lime juice
- 2 tbsp canola oil
- 1 medium carrot, sliced
- 1 small red bell pepper, sliced
- A pinch of salt and pepper
- 1/2 cup bean sprouts

Directions

1. Cook the rice according to package directions.

2. In a small mixing bowl, combine hoisin sauce, lime juice and 1 tablespoon water. Mix well and set aside.
3. On a large skillet add 1 tablespoon oil and heat over medium heat. Add the carrots and bell pepper and cook, stirring frequently, until tender, nearly 5 minutes. Transfer to a bowl.
4. Return the skillet to the stove, add another tablespoon of oil. Season the pork with salt and pepper and fry on a skillet, flipping couple times, Pour in the hoisin mixture and cook for 1 minute.
5. Return the vegetables to the skillet, add the bean sprouts (if using) and cook, tossing, until heated through, about 2 minutes. Serve over the rice and enjoy.

Classic Beef & Broccoli

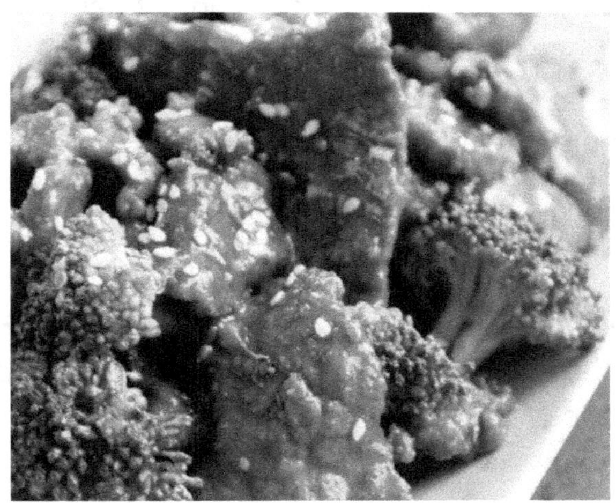

- Prep time: 25 minutes
- Cook time: 25 minutes
- Calories: 412

Ingredients

- 1/2 pound pork steak, halved lengthwise, then very thinly sliced crosswise
- 1 cup broccoli, cut into small florets
- 2 tbsp low-sodium soy sauce
- 4 tsp rice vinegar
- 2 cloves garlic, minced
- 1 tbsp brown sugar
- 1 tsp grated fresh ginger
- 1 tsp cornstarch
- 1 tbsp canola oil
- 1 small red chili, thinly sliced
- 2 scallions, thinly sliced

Directions

1. In a mixing bowl combine soy sauce and vinegar, add minced garlic. Add the meat and set aside for 5-10 minutes.
2. Place broccoli in a large skillet, add some water and simmer until nearly tender and bright green. Transfer to a plate.
3. Meanwhile, in another bowl mix together sugar, ginger, cornstarch, some soy sauce and vinegar, couple tbsp water.
4. Add the oil to a skillet and heat. Add beef in one layer and cook for 1-2 minutes. Add the sauce and simmer until meat will be tender. Add the broccoli and scallions and toss to combine.
5. Serve with or without rice.

Cod with Green Beans

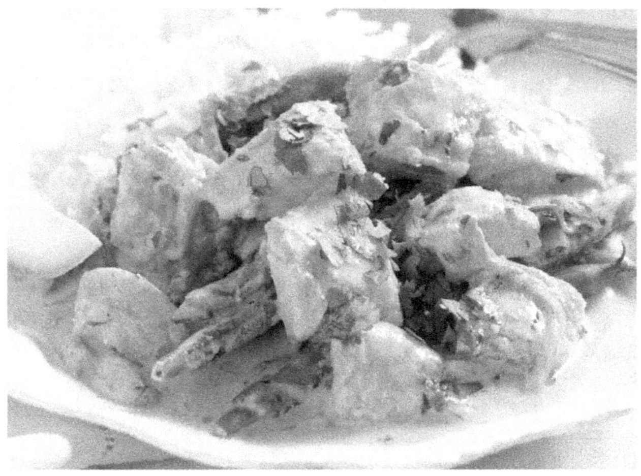

- Prep time: 5 minutes
- Cook time: 20 minutes
- Calories: 240

Ingredients

- 2 cod fillets
- 1/2 pound green beans
- 2 tbsp olive oil
- 1/4 cup Parmesan, grated
- 2 tbsp basil pesto
- Salt and pepper to taste

Directions

1. Preheat the oven to 420 F. Place beans on a large baking sheet, sprinkle with olive oil, season with salt and pepper, sprinkle with grated Parmesan. Roast until golden for about 10 minutes.

2. While cooking, preheat the large skillet with 1 tbsp oil. Season the cod with salt and pepper and fry fish from both sides until golden for about 2-4 minutes.
3. Spoon the pesto over the cod and serve with the beans.

Tilapia with Zoodles

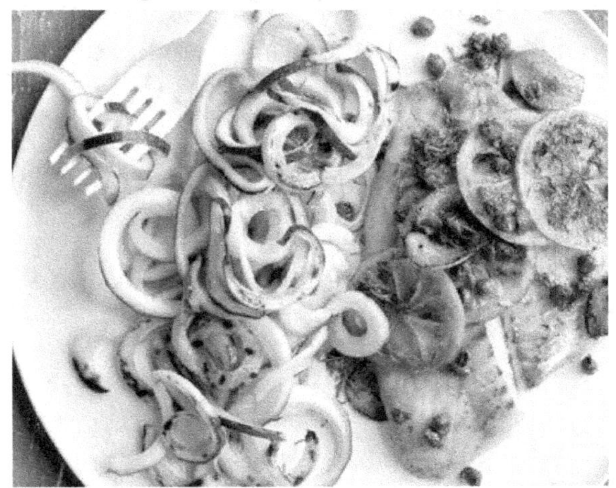

- Prep time: 10 minutes
- Cook time: 20 minutes
- Calories: 287

Ingredients

- 1 medium-sized zucchini, spiralized
- 2 medium tilapia fillets
- 3 tbsp olive oil
- 1/2 lemon, sliced
- 2 garlic cloves, chopped
- 1 tbsp capers (if desired)
- Freshly chopped parsley for garnish

Directions

1. Preheat the oven to 450 F. Take a baking sheet and place spiralized zucchini. Sprinkle with the olive oil and season with salt and pepper. Cook until tender and lightly golden for about 8-10 minutes.

2. While cooking, preheat the large skillet with 1 tablespoon olive oil on a medium heat. Season tilapia fillets with salt and pepper from both sides and fry for 3-5 minutes, until ready. Transfer to a plate.
3. Add 1 tbsp olive oil, then lemon, garlic, capers, and cook for couple minutes, stirring occasionally, for 2-4 minutes.
4. Serve fish, zoodles and lemon mixture, garnish with freshly chopped parsley and enjoy.

Chicken Fillets Marinated in Yogurt

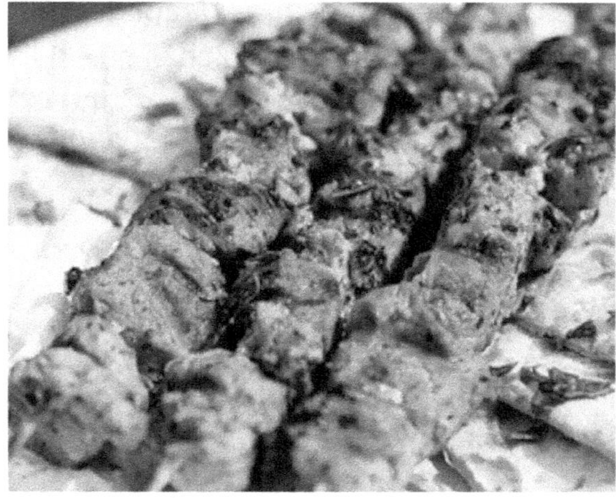

- Prep time: 30 minutes
- Cook time: 30 minutes
- Calories: 398

Ingredients

- 1 pound chicken breasts, boneless and skinless, cubed into 2-inch pieces
- 1/2 cup non-fat yogurt
- 2 garlic cloves, minced
- 1 tbsp grated ginger
- 1/2 tsp curry powder
- 1 tbsp lemon zest, grated
- 2 tbsp lemon juice
- 1 large bell pepper cut into 2-inch pieces
- 1 tbsp oil
- Salt and pepper to taste

Directions

1. In a large mixing bowl, combine the yogurt, garlic, ginger, curry powder, lemon zest, 2 tablespoons lemon juice. Season with salt and pepper and stir to combine. Add chicken cubes and set aside for 15 minutes.
2. Preheat your grill to medium-high. Thread the chicken and peppers onto skewers. Lightly oil the grill and cook the kebabs, turning couple times, until cooked through, 8 to 10 minutes.
3. Serve with rice, couscous or vegetables.

Spicy Lamb with Veggies

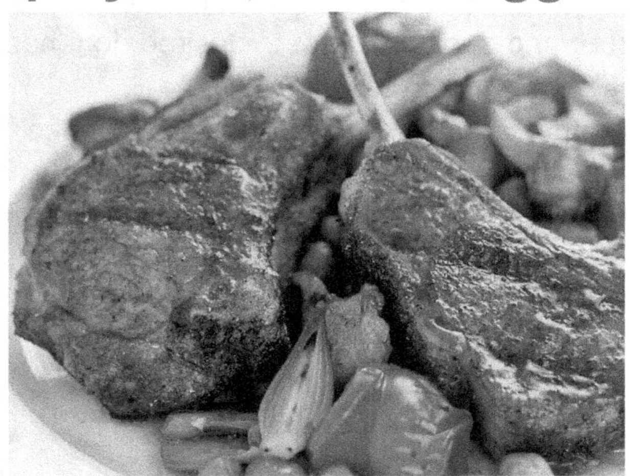

- Prep time: 20 minutes
- Cook time: 20 minutes
- Calories: 341

Ingredients

- 4 small lamb chops
- 2 medium-sized carrots
- 5 large radishes
- 3 tbsp olive oil
- 2 tbsp red wine vinegar
- 1/2 tsp honey
- 1/2 tsp ground cumin
- A pinch of salt and pepper

Directions

1. In a medium mixing bowl combine oil, vinegar, honey, cumin, season salt and pepper, and whisk to combine well. Set aside.

2. Preheat the skillet over medium-high heat. Sprinkle with tbsp of olive oil. Season the lamb chops with salt and pepper and cook on skillet to desired doneness - 4-6 minutes from each side.
3. While frying, use a vegetable peeler to make thin carrot strips and thin radish slices. Transfer veggies to a large bowl and cover with vinegar mixture. Combine well and serve with cooked lamb chops.

Pork Medallions with Herbs

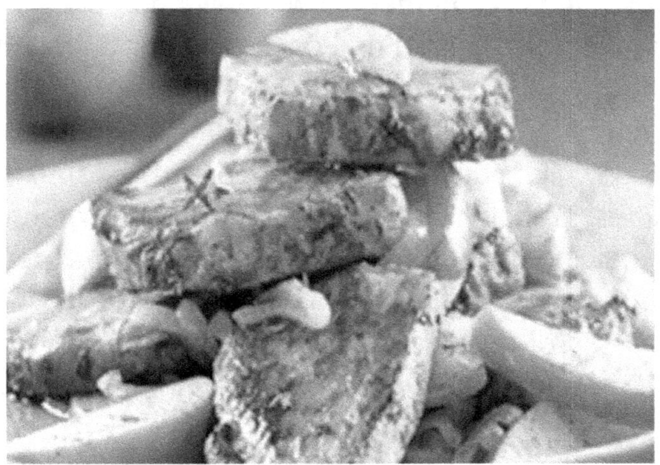

- Prep time: 20 minutes
- Cook time: 35 minutes
- Calories: 276

Ingredients

- 1 pound pork tenderloin
- 2 medium-sized carrots
- 1/2 pound asparagus
- 2 tbsp olive oil
- 1/2 cup freshly chopped parsley
- 1/2 tsp dried rosemary
- 1 package baby greens and herbs
- A pinch of salt and pepper

Directions

1. In a bowl combine chopped parsley and rosemary. Rub this mixture over the tenderloin and set aside.
2. Boil carrots for 5 minutes, chill. Do the same with asparagus for 3 minutes, until bright green and crisp.

3. Preheat oven to 380 F.
4. Cover the pork tenderloin with salt and pepper, preheat the ovenproof skillet and cook meat for 5-8 minutes until brown. Transfer to an oven and cook until ready and tender.
5. Meanwhile, cut carrots and asparagus into 2-inch-long sticks. Transfer to a large bowl, add baby greens, and remaining parsley. Season with salt and pepper and add remaining tablespoon oil. Add balsamic vinegar and stir to combine. Divide salad among serving plates.
6. Slice pork tenderloin and serve on the top of the salads.

Conclusion

Thank you again for downloading my cookbook! I Hope this book helps you to know more interesting and tasty recipes or inspire you to create your own unique dishes.

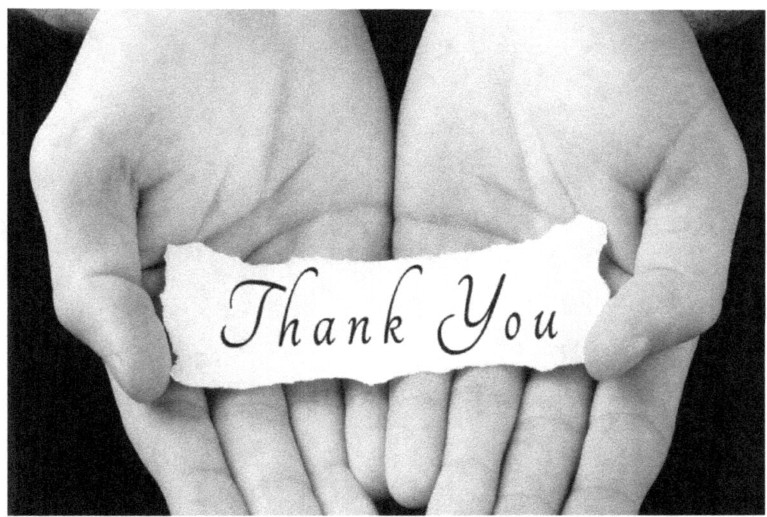